So, you think you want to be a nurse?

Catherine Prato-Lefkowitz PhD, MBA, MSN, RN

TABLE OF CONTENTS

SO, YOU THINK YOU WANT TO BE A NURSE?

Let me put this out there first. As a nurse educator, advocate, and one who has passion for nursing students, I've created a tool to help you connect the dots in nursing. Nursing can be overwhelming, but this tool will be your BFF (I promise)!

www.nursemuse.com

Great job on taking the first step toward becoming a nurse. Some people say they felt nursing was their "calling" and others found the passion for caring for others later in life. Nursing is a diverse career with so many options once you graduate! Before we talk about graduating, let's start from the beginning.

There are many different levels of nursing. All healthcare professionals are part of the healthcare team and each person on the team has vital roles to play. Let's talk about who is on the team.

The first, and most important person on the team is the patient. The patient is always the center of the team circle. Patients have a right to choose the types of care they receive and the procedures they would like and not like to have. The patient is the one who directs the team so the team members can create an individualized plan of care for that patient.

Another important team member is the medical provider. Depending on the patient's status he may have more than one provider who specializes in different areas of medicine. For example, the patient might have a cardiologist as well as a primary care doctor. The provider can be a medical doctor (MD or DO), an Advanced Practice Registered Nurse (APRN), or a Physician Assistant (PA). These professionals have training in assessing and diagnosing patients. Their role is to correctly diagnose the patient, order the correct diagnostic tests, correctly interpret test results, and prescribe appropriate medications and treatments.

Another important team member is the Certified Nursing Assistant (CNA). A CNA is a person who has gone to school and passed a state examination to obtain a certification as a nursing assistant. The CNA is a vital team member because the CNA will most likely see your patients more than you will! CNAs have scopes of practice that they must work within. This means there are tasks CNAs can and can't do. It is the nurse's responsibility to know the scope of practice for the CNA so that tasks are not delegated outside of the CNAs scope.

We keep talking about a scope of practice. What is that? Each state has a Nurse Practice Act. Within the Nurse Practice Act are statutes and regulations that give certified and licensed medical personnel a scope to work within. CNAs, nurses, physicians, respiratory therapists, physical therapists, pharmacists, and all of the other medical professionals are not legally allowed to work outside of their scope of practice. So, before you get accepted into nursing school, make sure to go to your state's Board of Nursing website and download their Nurse Practice Act.

The next team member we will discuss is the nurse. When I say nurse, know there are different levels of education within nursing. There are Licensed Practical Nurses, Associate Degree Nurses, and a Bachelor of Science in Nursing. A Licensed Practical Nurse (LPN) has gone to school for about 18 months and passed the NCLEX-PN examination and holds a license as an LPN. Again, LPNs have a scope of practice! An Associate Degree Nurse (AND) has gone to a two-year college and taken their NCLEX-RN examination and holds a license as a Registered Nurse (RN). A Bachelor of Science of Nursing (BSN) RN is a nurse who has received a bachelor's degree from a four-year university and has taken and passed the NCLEX-RN. You may ask what the difference between an ADN and a BSN is if they both hold an RN license. The answer is that a BSN degree not only teaches the different areas of nursing, but also places emphasis on leadership, scholarship, and evidence-based practice.

Other important team members include physical therapists, occupational therapists, social workers, speech therapists, and environmental services (just to name a few). It is amazing how many people are on the patient's team to help him regain his optimal ability. Let's talk about why nursing is one of the best professions out there!

WHY IS NURSING A GREAT PROFESSION?

Congratulations on thinking about becoming a nurse. This book is designed to help you become familiar with the requirements nursing school will place on you. Every school may be a little different, but one thing is the same and that is nursing school requires a lot of hard work, a lot of time, and much dedication. Nursing school is challenging, but in the end it is worth it.

Why is nursing a great PROFESSION? I highlight the word **profession** because nursing has evolved into a highly-skilled, technical, evidence-based profession. 50 years ago, nurses were not required to have the education, skills, medical and nursing knowledge, and technical knowledge that nurses must have today! It has changed drastically. Hospitals and facilities could not function without the nurses. This is both and good and a bad thing!

Nurses are being required to take on more responsibility than ever before. Not only do you need to care for patients, but you will be required to know every detail about every medication you give, every detail about every procedure your patient is scheduled to have, every potential sign and symptom of a poor outcome from that procedure, every change in each of your patients' status. You must be organized so you can care for 6 patients at a time, know each patient's diagnosis, medications, status, provider, and family members! On top of this you must know who the other nurses are on the unit, who is off the unit with a patient, your roll in a code for that day, know who is on lunch, who called off, who is covering who, and where the nursing students and residents are and what they can and cannot do in terms of skills—and keep a smile on your face and remain calm! It sounds overwhelming, but it is fun. I promise.

I just want you to know you are entering a profession. This begins from day one of nursing school. You need to treat your professors and the other students with respect. The other day a faculty member shared with me that he received an email from a student, and it started out "Hey Dude, what are we supposed to read this week?" This did not end well for the student, and it upset the faculty member. Be respectful when speaking to, and with, your faculty. Call the faculty by their professional titles, be professional in your email communication, be professional in the classroom (raise your hand), show up on time (early), be prepared, and be open and willing to learn. You might not like all your faculty members, but they are there to teach you and most of them have many, many years of experience!

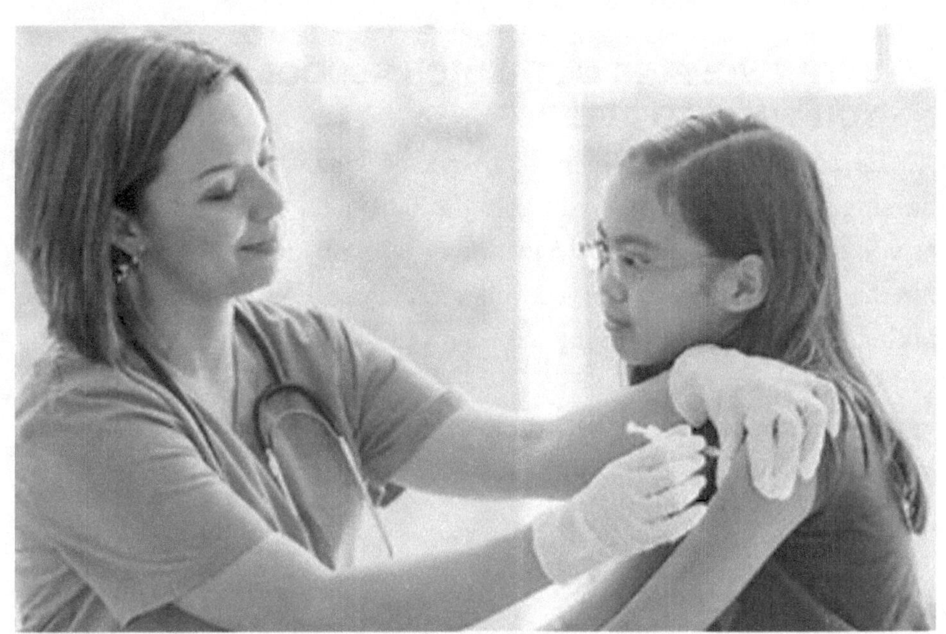

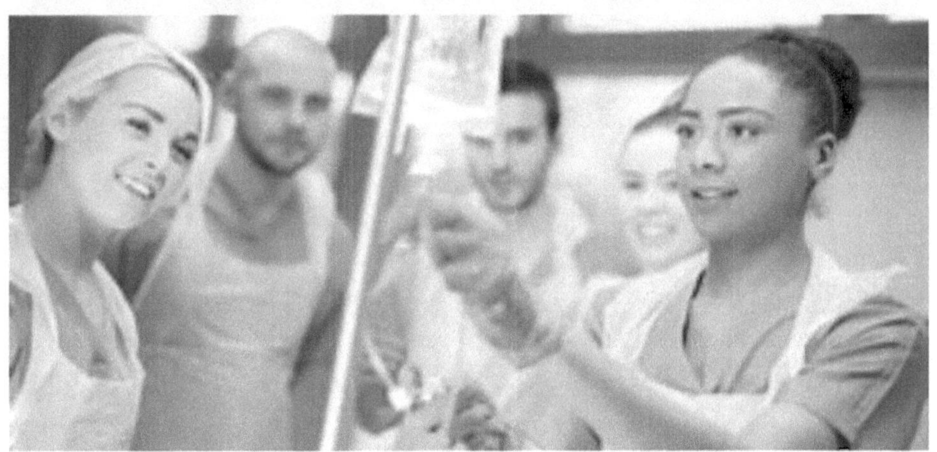

✓ STEP ONE: DECIDE TO GO TO NURSING SCHOOL

✓ STEP TWO: FIND OUT WHICH SCHOOL YOU WANT TO ATTEND.

Here is where you will need to decide where you will begin your nursing school career. Are you going to become an LPN and then work as you continue toward your ADN or BSN? Are you going to go straight for the BSN? This is what you must decide so you do not waste time taking extra classes or missing out on classes that are offered only during certain semesters.

Regardless of which path you take there are prerequisite classes that are pretty much universal for the medical professions.

Plan on taking:
- English
- Math
- History
- Humanities and Fine Arts
- Social Sciences
- Life and Physical Sciences
- Chemistry
- Anatomy and Physiology

Make sure you contact an advisor at the school before registering for any classes so she can help you map out your plan of study. Remember, there are many students trying to get into nursing school so there will be a large list of students needing to take the same classes as you. An advisor can help you get registered early and can tell you the sequence in which to take the courses.

✓ STEP THREE: DETERMINE THE PROGRAM YOU WANT TO GO FOLLOW AND MEET WITH AN ADVISOR.

As soon as you choose which school you are going to, make a phone call and get an advisor. Tell the advisor you want to go to nursing school, and you need a plan of study.

Here are some questions to ask:

- Can we meet to plan my class schedule?
- What sequence should I take the prerequisites in?
- Are there any prerequisites offered in the summer session?
- How do I go about getting permission to enter a class if it is full when I try to register?
- When should I plan on officially making my major Nursing?

Questions you have to ask yourself before starting your classes:

- Do I have to work?
- If I must work, how many hours do I have to work to pay my bills?
- Are there ways to change my work schedule so I can attend school and meet all of the requirements?
- How am I going to pay for college?
- How am I going to save money, so I don't have to work while in nursing school?
- What scholarships can I apply for through the college or university?

✓ STEP FOUR: MAKE A PLAN AND STICK TO IT

Now that you have your schedule and know what classes you need to take and when to take them, you need to focus on getting the best grades you can. Many nursing schools are competitive and grades in the prerequisites are taken into consideration of who gets in. Understand that for every three-hour class you take you will need to devote nine hours a week to studying for that class. Use a calendar to plan out your semester. Identify when you will go to school, when you will study, and when you will work. Make sure the plan is reasonable and something you can stick to. Prerequisites will take about two years for a BSN program and about one year for an ADN program. Be prepared to use all your spare time studying. This will prepare you for nursing school!

If you find yourself falling behind or having a hard time, call your advisor. Talk to your advisor and see if there can be a change to your plan. If you are having a hard time in a class, email your professor. Professors want students to be successful. Communicate with your professors. Ask questions if you have questions. Clarify if something is not clear. Highlight all your deadlines for papers and tests and quizzes on your calendar.

✓ STEP FIVE: APPLY TO NURSING SCHOOL

You are going to apply to the program. You want to go to the Board of Nursing website and find the school's NCLEX pass rate. You want to attend a program that has a high pass rate, one that is not in trouble with the Board of Nursing, and has a positive reputation in the community.

You are coming to an end with your prerequisites and your advisor has told you how to officially make your major Nursing! It is now time to throw your hat into the ring to become a nurse. This is exciting!

Know that getting into nursing school is competitive! Make sure you have high grades in all your prerequisites. Be prepared to write a statement on why you want to become a nurse. Be prepared for a possible face-to-face interview. Be prepared to take an entry placement test!

Questions to think about when writing a personal statement or sitting for an interview:

- Why do I want to be a nurse?
- What medical experience have I had (volunteering, CNA, EMT, etc.)?

- How do I plan on being successful in nursing school knowing that it will be an 80–90-hour weekly commitment for one to two years?
- Do I have reliable transportation to get to clinicals and class on time?
- Do I have a support system to be there to help me when I need help?
- Am I 100% committed to putting in the hard work to become a nurse?
- What life experiences can I use to demonstrate I have critical thinking skills?
- What life experiences can I use to demonstrate I am a clear communicator?
- When have I been on a team and how do I act when on a team (leader, follower)?
- What will I bring to the nursing profession?
- What are my goals after graduating?

If you must take an entrance exam, the nursing program will let you know which test you will take. Most likely it will be the HESI or the TEAS. Once you find out which test it is, buy a study guide to prepare. The test score will determine your placement on "the list".

Usually nursing programs look at you as a whole. They take into consideration your grades, your previous medical experience, your written essay or interview, and the score on the entrance exam.

✓ STEP SIX : STARTING NURSING SCHOOL

Congratulations! You made it in. You are proud, your family is proud, and your friends are proud. Be excited and celebrate, but then get to work! From day one of nursing school, you must be 100% committed to doing what it takes to make it. Long are the days of striving for all as, truly, student nurses *strive* to make it to the next class. It is hard! Not that you can't do it, but just know it is challenging. It takes organization, support, and planning.

During your orientation day you will get to meet your cohort of students as well as the faculty and staff. Make sure you get to know everyone! The faculty will let you know the expectations of the program, the expectations regarding dress, and timeliness, etc. Ask many questions so everything is clear. Make sure to get to know your cohort! These are the people you will be practically living with for the next one to two years! Nursing school friends are friends you will have for life. You will laugh together, and cry together, and get to know one another very well!

Your nursing program will tell you when your classes are and where and when your clinicals are. This is why it is important to save money, so you do not have to work during nursing school. Again, apply for scholarships, apply for student aid, or ask your family for help!

Each semester or session you will be going to school on different days. Some clinicals are 12-hour clinicals during the day, and some are twelve-hour clinicals during the night. Some clinicals might be eight hours and some might be four. Just understand that every semester will be different days/hours/shifts that you must work around. You are required to attend all lectures, all clinicals, and all labs. Most programs allow one absence before dismissing students from the nursing program! Nursing school will also teach you that "early is the new on-time". All students are required to be in class, or lab, or clinicals at least 15 minutes early. This is a great life skill to have. When you are working as a nurse you will be expected to be on time to relieve the prior shift.

✓ STEP SIX B: SURVIVING NURSING SCHOOL

Be prepared to do a lot of paperwork before being officially accepted into nursing school. You will most likely need a physical exam, proof of health insurance, a TB test, and vaccination records. The program will tell you what is expected but be sure to give yourself time to get all requirements completed. If these requirements are not completed, you may not be allowed to enter a clinical facility, and this will cause you to be dropped from the program.

Nursing school will fly by. However, there is A LOT to learn in nursing school. From day one you will have hundreds of pages of textbooks to read, tests and quizzes to prepare for, papers to write, projects to complete, care plans to write, and homework to finish. Nursing school will teach you how to be a safe nurse. The goal of nursing school is to make you a safe, NOVICE nurse. Many people believe they should be an expert by the time they graduate, and this is not realistic. The NCLEX will test to ensure you are a SAFE nurse. People do not become experts in any field until they've accumulated about 10 years of experience. Nursing school will allow you to learn about different specialties so you can see what you might enjoy doing, but the goal is to learn the fundamentals and the basics to be SAFE.

Classes you will take in nursing school include Fundamentals of Nursing, Medical Surgical Nursing (usually 1-3 rotations), Obstetrical Nursing, Pediatric Nursing, Mental Health Nursing, and Community Nursing. Students usually get a chance to float to the Emergency Room, Operating Room, and other departments during their Medical Surgical clinicals, but it depends on the facility and the program. Each class builds upon the previous class so don't let the knowledge fly out of your brain after you pass the first semester or session. You will need to carry that knowledge from class to class so you can build upon it and develop critical thinking skills along the way.

Math... Math is fun! Ok, maybe not everyone thinks so. Math is essential in nursing because medication doses are based on math calculations. Pediatric medication dosages are based on weight. Math is important and most likely you will have a math test at the beginning of each course. The norm is three strikes, and you are out. This sounds harsh, but if you do not pass the math calculation tests you could potentially cause a fatal dosing error. Remember our job is to be SAFE. If you are nervous about math talk to your professors. Ask for tutoring, ask for help. There are many different methods of calculating dosages. You need to find the one that makes sense to you and practice, practice, practice.

Tests and quizzes in nursing school are different than what you are used to. Up until this point you have been tested on knowledge level questions. You are probably used to reading chapters and taking notes and doing well on exams. Nursing school questions are different. The questions will require you to use the knowledge you have and apply the knowledge to the question. Not only will you be required to apply the knowledge, but you will have multiple answer choices (meaning more than one answer) or choose the BEST answer (meaning all the answers are correct, but you choose the best one). It is possible, and you will make it by thinking critically and getting into the habit of asking yourself "why". As a nurse you must know the "why" behind everything you do!

You can get ahead of the game and search the NCSBN website to see the NCLEX-PN and NCLEX-RN test plans. The National Council of State Boards of Nursing (NCSBN) tells you what is on the NCLEX test. Well, they tell you the areas of concepts upon which you will be tested. Download the test blueprint. Use this as a study guide as you move through nursing school. Within the next year the NCSBN is introducing the Next Generation NCLEX which means their test questions will really delve into critical thinking and clinical judgment. The test will include drag and drop answers, diagrams, standard multiple-choice questions, and 'select all that apply' questions, to mention but a few. Keep this in mind as you study throughout nursing school. When you study questions, it is always good to get the correct answer, but force yourself to understand why the other answers could be incorrect. The more you do this the more critical thinking you will be using!

Make sure you understand what type of learner you are. There are many self-assessments out there. Some people learn best by visual aids, others by auditory aids, others by writing. Be prepared to use your strengths when in lectures. Know how you will take notes. Will you type notes, or will you hand write them? Will you ask permission to record a lecture so you can listen to it while driving? Will you have a study buddy and share and compare notes? Will you find a few classmates and have scheduled study sessions? Be prepared ahead of time so you are prepared to succeed! Like it was noted before, you must have a schedule and a calendar and plan out your days, so you aren't reading 500 pages the night before a lecture.

When you go into clinical settings remember you are the guest of the facility. This means you must act professionally, do as the facility asks in terms of parking, placing lunch boxes, sitting, etc. There are so many nursing schools trying to get into clinical sites that it can sometimes get dirty! Any time a nursing program does not comply with a clinical site's expectations or requests the program can be asked not to return. You do not want to be in the cohort that got kicked out of a clinical site! If you have an issue or a problem with a clinical site, you should always direct your concerns to your faculty member.

Speaking of clinical sites... Some units will welcome you and your clinical group with open arms. Some nurses LOVE to teach and will want to show you everything and have you practice as many skills as you can. Other units might not be so welcoming. Some nurses do not want a student that day (and this is fine). Just tell your faculty member that you need to work with another nurse. Remember the nurses are there to work. Having a student on top of their patient load might be too much for them. Do not take it personally. This happens sometimes. If you are with a nurse who does not want to "teach" then just make sure to communicate with the nurse what you will and will not be doing. If you are assigned one of the nurse's patients for the day you can say "I will be doing the morning assessment on patient X, I am not able to document in the electronic medical record, but I will write down my assessment on a piece of paper and give it to you, I will pass medications for this patient with my instructor and let you know when I am finished with all of that." This way you are not "in the way" and the nurse knows what you are doing and how you will communicate with her. Nurses will appreciate you taking the bull by the horns. Nurses watch to see which students are the go-getters and which ones are trying to hide. Think of every clinical rotation as a job interview. Many nursing students get their first job at a unit they worked on during nursing school because they worked hard, asked a lot of questions, took initiative, and was noticed by the unit's manager or director!

Seek out opportunities. Many hospitals these days offer Nurse Apprentice Programs (NAP). These NAP positions are paid positions for nursing students to work on a unit as a NAP. The student nurse can perform skills they have been checked off on by their faculty. NAP positions are competitive, but if you are fortunate to be hired as a NAP, it is getting your foot in the door to be hired as a nurse after passing the NCLEX. These positions are great because they pay you and the hospital understands that you are in nursing school, so you are only required to work 2-3 shifts per month. Some hospitals even allow you to do half a shift! NAPs are placed in all departments—from the Emergency Room to the NICU to Maternity. Again, you will need to interview and be in good standing with your nursing program, but this is a great way to gain more clinical experience before graduating.

Many hospitals are also offering new graduate programs where the new graduates are placed with an experienced nurse for months to work with that nurse and learn the flow of the hospital. These programs also offer lectures and simulation classes for new graduates to help them assimilate into their new role as a nurse.

Bottom line is that there are many opportunities that will allow you to learn as much as you want to learn. You must keep your eyes and ears open and be willing to sign up for experiences, even if you are nervous (that is normal).

Many programs have a Student Nurses Association (SNA). This is a good organization to become involved with. The SNA usually holds many different activities such as health fairs, blood drives, or food donations, etc. Again, this is another way to get known in the program. Once the faculty see you are going above and beyond you put yourself in a position to receive scholarships or opportunities to attend conferences that others might not be invited to.

Remember how I said earlier that for every three hours of class you will need nine hours of study time? This holds true for nursing school as well. Many traditional programs have students taking four classes at one time. Other programs have shorter sessions, but have the students take one to two classes at a time. Again, these are questions you should be asking the program you are interested in attending. You want to be successful, so you need to choose a program that fits your learning style and your life!

School can be overwhelming, and this is where your cohort friends come in. Your classmates are going through the same thing. I told you earlier you will laugh, and you will cry with your friends. I did not lie. Some days you might need to go sit at a coffee shop and complain about how hard nursing school is. Sometimes you might need an ear to listen to how you felt "dumb" for not knowing an answer on a test. This is all normal! Everyone needs support in nursing school. This is why it is important to make friends and have a group who can understand the stress you are feeling because they are feeling it too! After your pity party you can pick yourself up and get back to studying!

✓ STEP SEVEN: APPLYING FOR THE NCLEX

Great job: you finished nursing school. Now you get to apply for the NCLEX. This is the time you need to go to the Board of Nursing website for the state you are getting your initial nursing license in and apply. There are different requirements for different states. You must complete their application, pay the fees, get your fingerprints done (fingerprints can take up to 6 months to get processed), send your transcripts to the Board of Nursing, apply to Pearson Vue to sit for the NCLEX, pay Pearson Vue and wait for your Authorization to Test (ATT). You will not receive your ATT until the Board of Nursing has verified that you have graduated from nursing school. If you happen to have any criminal history, you must gather all of the court paperwork demonstrating the case is closed and that you are in good standing. Some Boards of Nursing might require a letter from you stating what occurred that caused this issue with the law and how you have grown and why they should grant you a nursing license. If you have any question about a criminal history, you should contact the Board of Nursing before applying to nursing school to make sure you will be able to receive a nursing license. After all the paperwork has been signed off, you will be able to schedule your NCLEX test date. You only need to take the NCLEX once, —once you pass you can endorse your license into other states. Each state has their own application process and requirements, but you only need to pass the NCLEX once.

 ## STEP EIGHT: KEEPING YOUR NURSING LICENSE IN GOOD STANDING AND GETTING INVOLVED

Congratulations. You passed the NCLEX. Now, part of being a professional is keeping your nursing license in good standing. Check with your Board of Nursing to see when you need to renew your license. Each state has their own renewal cycle. Each state also has their own continuing education requirements you must complete before renewing your license. The worst thing you can do is forget to renew your nursing license because then you can be disciplined by the Board of Nursing for practicing without a license! Read the Board of Nursing renewal requirements before it is time to renew. Know what is expected. Some states require fingerprints every six years, and some states are every eight years. Boards of Nursing can do random audits when nurses renew their license. Normally when you renew your license you attest you did the correct amount of continuing education, and if audited you are required to submit proof of this. If you are unable to provide proof, you might find yourself in front of the Board of Nursing. Read the Board of Nursing website frequently as ignorance is not an excuse in the eyes of the Board. Stay up to date with Board rule changes, requirement changes, statute changes, and regulation changes.

Once you feel comfortable in your new role as a nurse you can apply to be on the Board of Nursing committees. Boards of Nursing have committees where practicing nurses can work with the Board to make changes to rules. Some committees include the Education Advisory Committee, and the APRN committee. This is a great way to serve your nursing community and to network and meet more nurses in your community. Boards of Nursing usually put out a quarterly magazine or newsletter and they are always looking for articles. Submit articles for publication that pertain to nursing regulation or legislation.

✓ STEP NINE: STARTING YOUR CAREER

Let's begin with what options are out there for nurses and then we will discuss specifics.

There are many opportunities within nursing. You have probably heard this from many people. Nursing is a career where one need never get bored. Once you are successful and pass your licensing exam you should

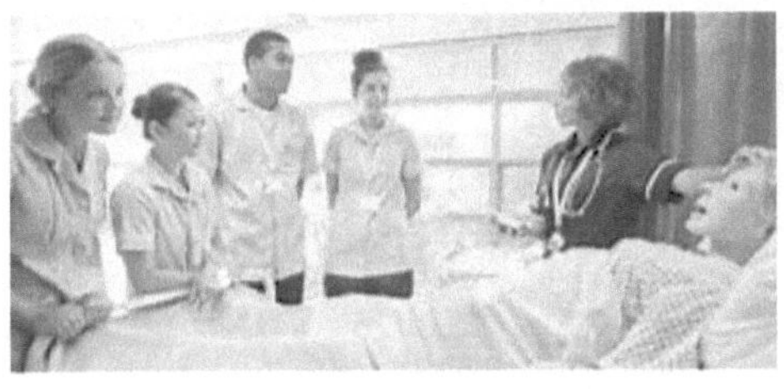
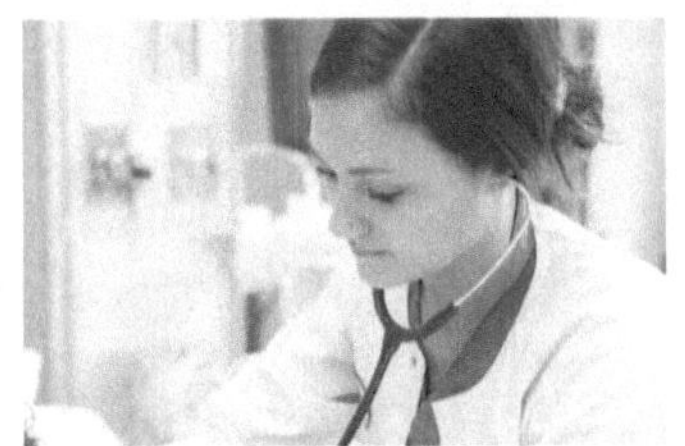

spend some time working in a hospital to really get your foundational skills solidified. After you spend a couple of years working in a hospital and gain some experience, the opportunities are endless.

We are in a time where many more nurses will be needed soon. Much of the nursing demographic is getting close to retirement age and there will be a gap to fill. As you may know, patients are living longer, have more acute illnesses and are requiring more time in the hospital. Between the aging population living longer and many nurses looking to retire, there will be a need for many more nurses, very soon.

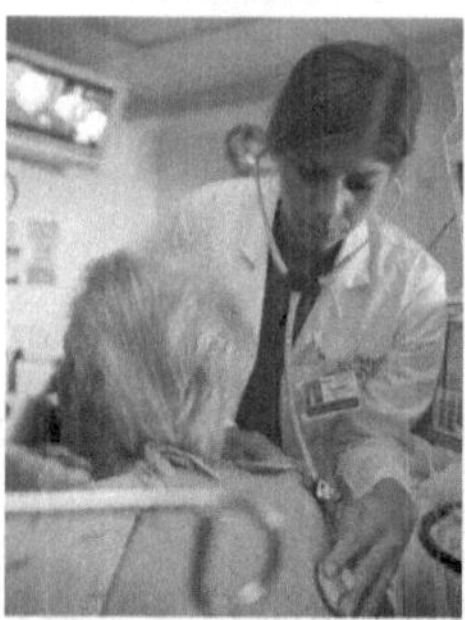

There is also a push these days to increase the number of insured patients so patients can receive health care. With more people insured there will be more patients to see. This also contributes to the need for more nurses.

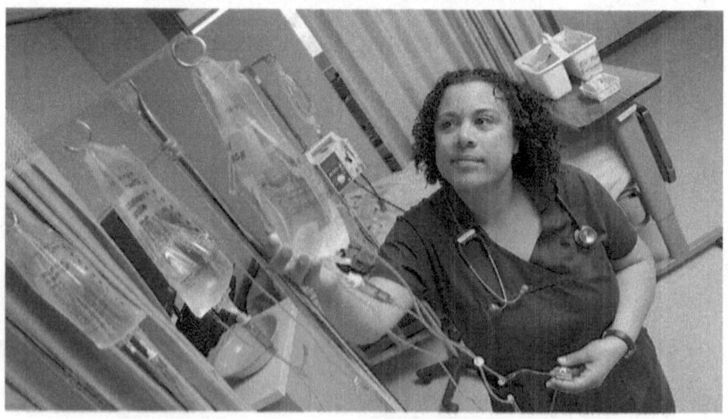

So, as you can see there are many reasons why nurses will be needed in the future.

WHAT ARE THE CHARACTERISTICS OF A NURSE?

What are some characteristics of a nurse? You probably want to be a nurse because you want to help people, but do you know what it really takes to be a nurse? Here are some common characteristics of nurses:

Caring: Nurses must be caring. You probably think this should not have to be mentioned, but caring is the heart of our profession. Caring does not mean feeling empathy for the patient and wanting to help them, although this is important as well. Caring means you are competent and knowledgeable. This means you will really have to study and know the material. You will be working on the front lines of healthcare once you are a nurse, and it comes down to you knowing what to do in different situations to provide the best quality care you can. Caring means missing your lunch to sit with a patient who is scared. Caring is staying late to help the night shift who are short staffed. Caring is being an advocate for your patient when they feel no one is listening to their needs.

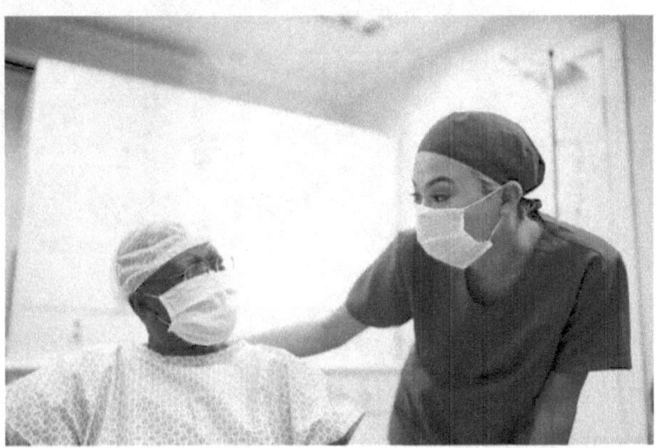

You must be able to **critically think.** Nursing school will help you develop your critical thinking skills, but this is crucial to nursing. Every day you will be challenged with situations you must critically think through. Not every patient is the same and not every patient needs the same treatment plan or interventions; it is up to you to critically think and analyze how to best care for different patients.

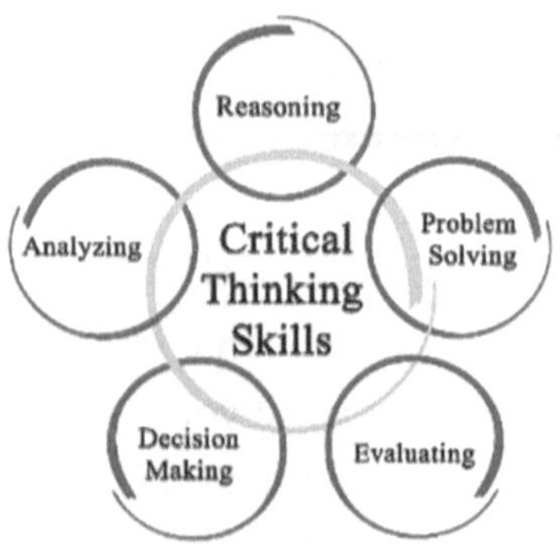

You must **follow through** with what you say you will do. Building a trusting relationship is paramount in nursing. Nurses have consistently been rated one of the top professions people trust. We **build this trust** by being open and honest with our patients. We build this trust by following through on what we tell our patients. If you tell your patient you will come into the room the next morning to check on them then you must follow through.

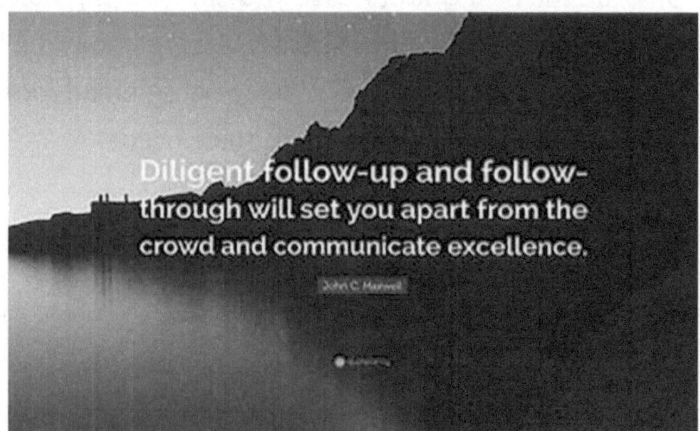

To be a caring nurse you must work 100% for your patients and their families and make sure their care is **patient-centered**. You must get to know your patients and their wishes so you may relay this information to the other healthcare team members. The patient is at the center of the healthcare team and nurses work as their advocates to ensure their needs are being met; physically as well as psychologically.

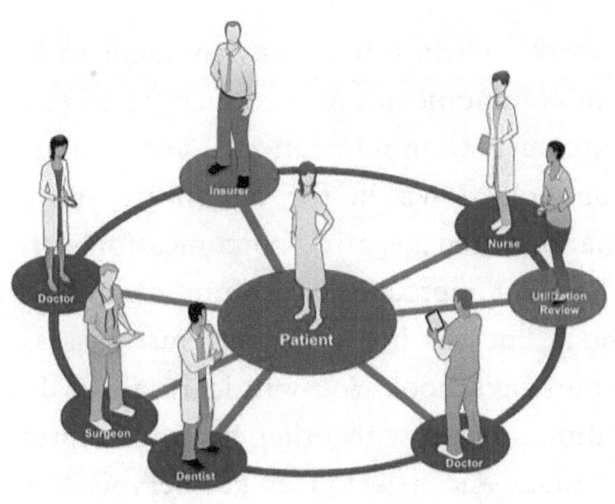

You must know the most **current research** about your area of work so you provide the best evidence-based care you can. Hopefully you enjoy reading. Nursing school is filled with reading. You will be reading many professional nursing journals. You will be reading journal articles, analyzing them, and using what you learn and incorporate it at the bedside. Nursing is driven by evidence-based, scholarly work. The only way to keep up on the most current literature is to read it.

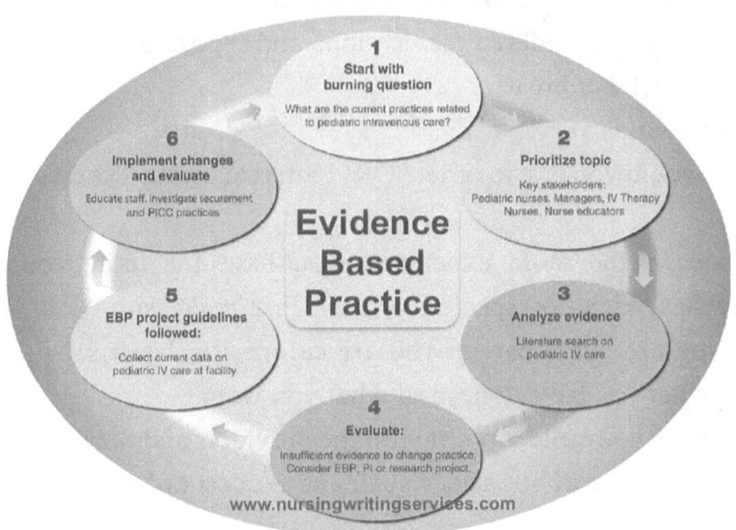

You must work well in a team environment so everyone on the healthcare team communicates and cooperates to ensure the patient has the best outcomes. Communication is very important in nursing. Communication breakdown in the healthcare setting can lead to unplanned, unanticipated negative outcomes for your patients. You will be taught the best approaches to communicating effectively while you are in school, but this is a skill you must possess prior to being admitted to a nursing school. You will learn about different types of ways nurses communicate with other healthcare professionals. One thing student nurses and new nurses get nervous about is calling a provider for an order or to tell her about a status change. When you must make your first few calls make a list of what you will say. Here is a template:

Hello this is nurse X calling from Summerlin Hospital floor 3 West.

I am calling about your patient Jane Doe who was admitted last night for COPD exacerbation.

Her current vital signs are X, Y, Z (blood pressure, pulse, respiration, temperature, oxygen saturation).

She is complaining of shortness of breath.

I have given the ordered medications and repositioned her, but she is not able to catch her breath.

Breath sounds are X, Y, Z.

What would you like to order? OR, I am requesting a chest X-Ray and an SVN.

Of course, the more experience you have the more you will be comfortable asking for specific orders. Just make sure you are clear on who you are, what patient you are calling for, latest vital signs, the problem, what you have done, and what you want.

Also, once you build rapport with the providers and they are confident in your abilities it will be easier to call and request orders.

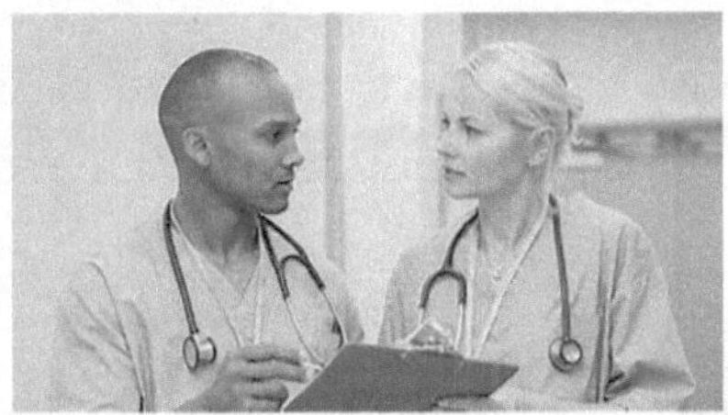
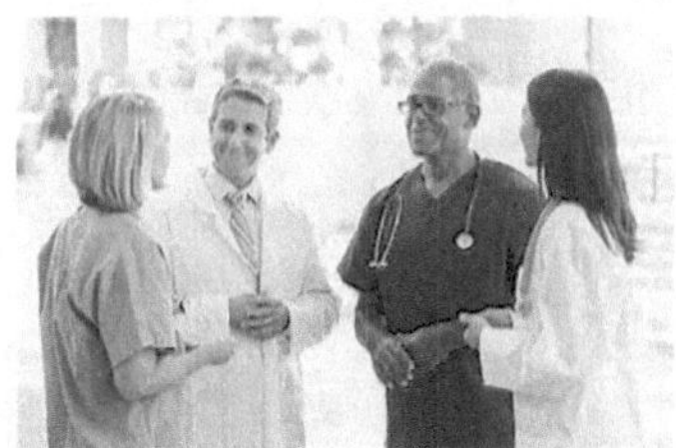

You must **be professional** and hold your profession in the highest regard. You will be the face of nursing when you interact with your patients, their families, and other healthcare workers. How you represent yourself is how others will "see" nursing. Being professional is top priority for our profession.

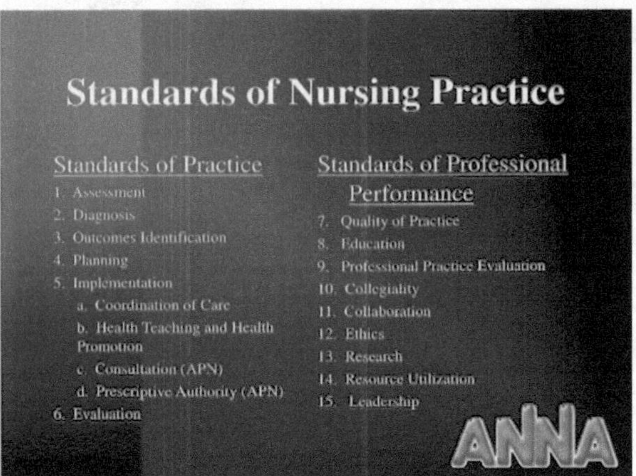

WHERE CAN I WORK AS A NURSE?

Where can you work after you graduate from nursing school and pass the licensing examination? There are many different areas to work within the nursing field. As mentioned above, nursing is a great career because there are so many opportunities for nurses.

There are many different practice settings nurses can work in. There are acute care settings such as hospitals. Within hospitals you have many different areas of specialties to choose from, such as Pediatrics, Labor and Delivery, Medical Surgical, and the Operating Room, just to mention a few.

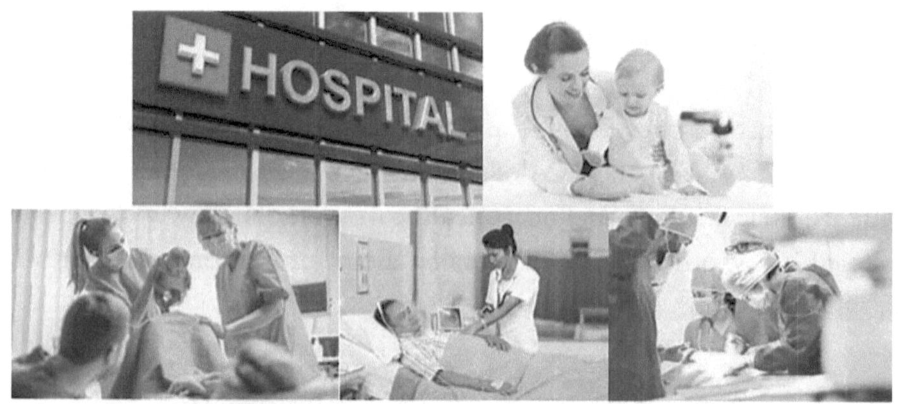

Nurses also work in ambulatory care settings. Examples of these would be outpatient surgery centers or outpatient clinics where the patients come to you for services and do not stay overnight.

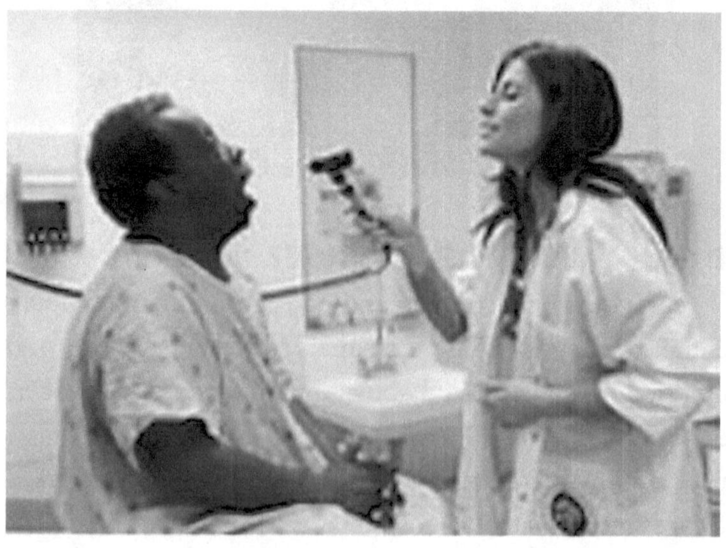

There are also opportunities for community health nursing positions. Examples of opportunities for community nursing would include hospice nurses, school nurses, public health nurses, and mental health outpatient nurses to mention a few.

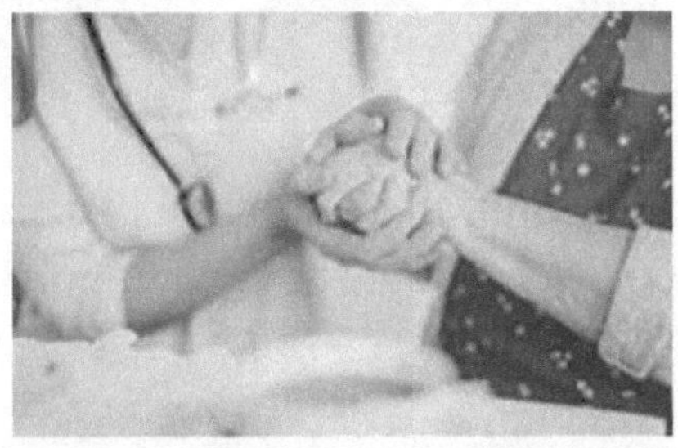
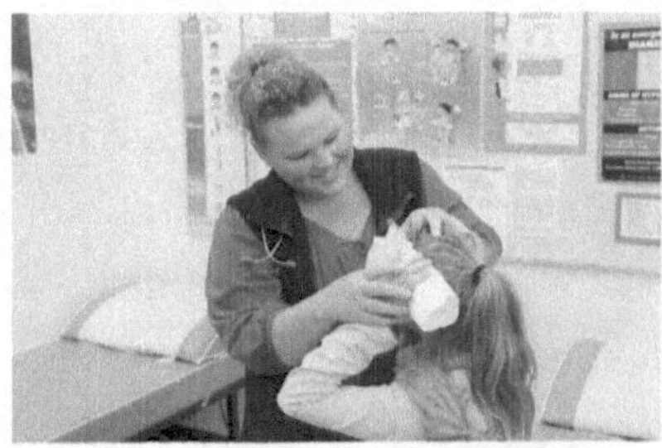

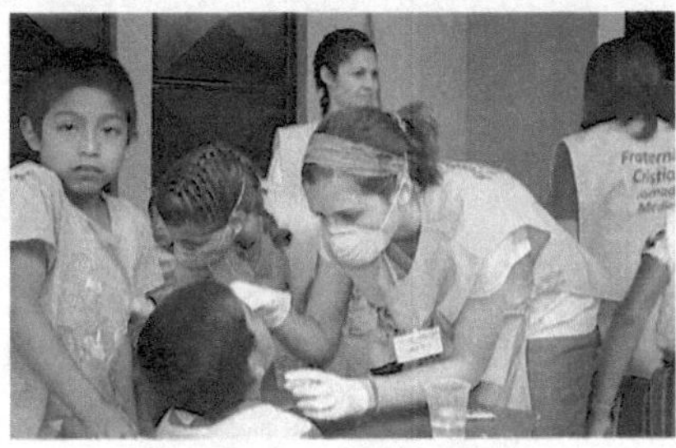
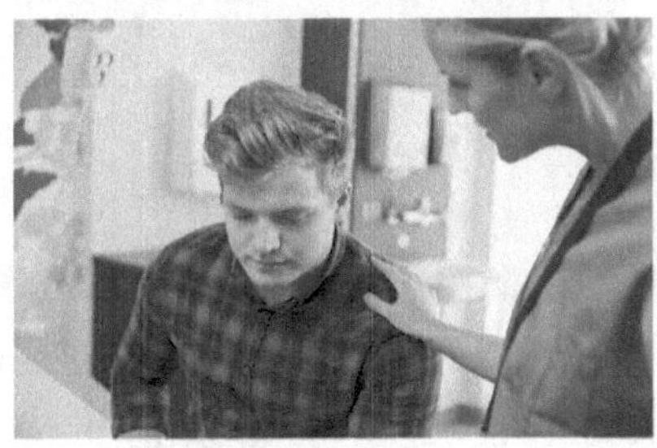

As mentioned above, most nurses work in the acute care settings for a few years before they move into a nursing specialty. Most students are advised to work on a general Medical Surgical floor for a couple of years before moving into a specialty. This is because you will gain a tremendous amount of experience on the Medical Surgical floor

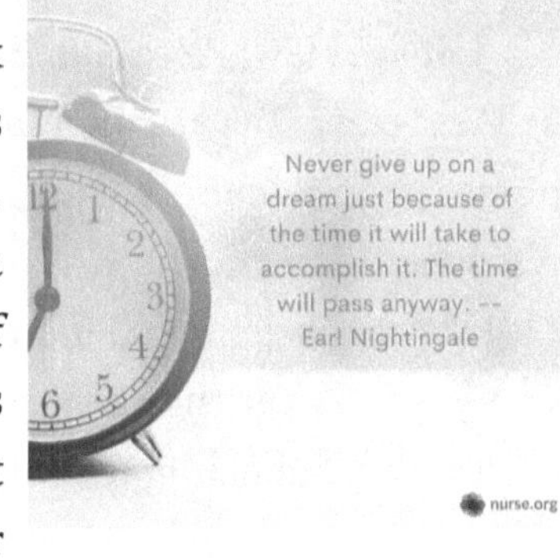

while solidifying your fundamental skills in nursing. Once you gain confidence and have experience with the general nursing aspect, then you will be able to move into a specialty area with ease.

While you are working to complete your nursing education, ask yourself which populations you enjoy working with. Just like the different areas of nursing you can work with; you can also tailor your nursing to specific populations. There are nurses who work with the elderly (Geriatrics), and there

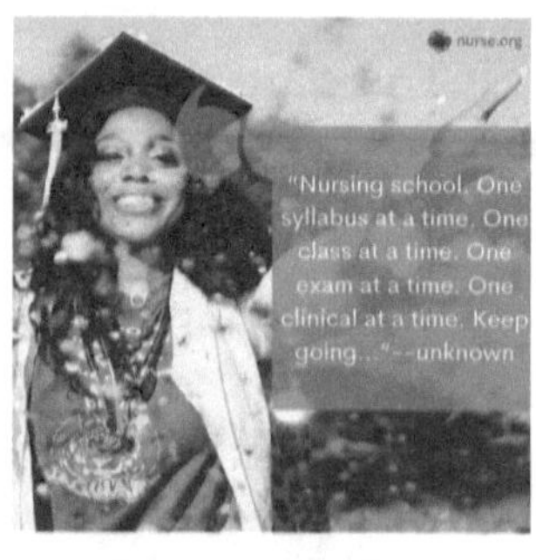

are nurses who work with children (Pediatrics), and then there are nurses who work with adults. Most nursing students come into nursing believing they know where they want to work. One great aspect of nursing school is it will introduce you to many aspects of nursing. You will do rotations on the General Medical Surgical floors, but you will also do rotations through other units and work with a variety of patient populations.

WHAT CAN I DO AFTER NURSING SCHOOL?

One wonderful aspect of nursing is the different levels of schooling it offers. Here is a breakdown of the levels of nursing:

Let's review: Associate Science Nurses (ASN) or Associate Degree in Nursing (ADN): These nurses go to a school where they will receive their Associate Science in Nursing OR an Associate Degree in Nursing. Generally, this takes about two years. After they complete their degree they sit for the licensing examination, the NCLEX and, after passing, they become Registered 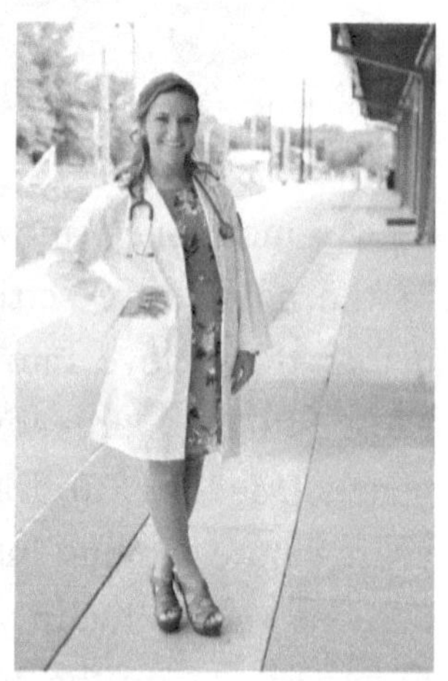 Nurses. There is a push across the country to have most nurses receive their BSN. Many people go to school and receive their ASN or ADN and take an RN to BSN completion program to receive their BSN degree while working as a nurse.

RN to BSN Program: These programs can be found online or onsite at most of the major universities. This program focuses on the non-clinical content the ADN does not provide during nursing school. Examples of classes that would be found in an RN to 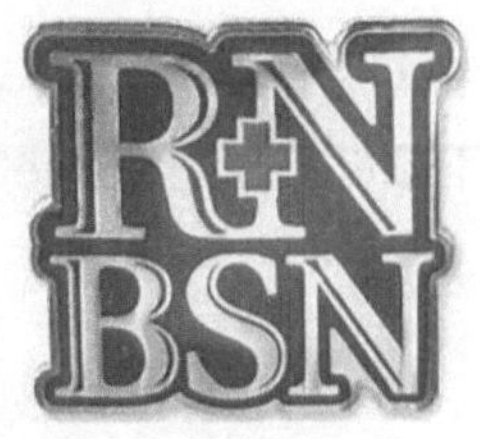 BSN curriculum would include Evidence Based Practice, Professional Nursing Issues, or Nursing Leadership. These are non-clinical courses that ASN and ADN nurses can take online or onsite and receive their BSN after successful completion.

Bachelor's Degree Nurses (BSN): These nurses go to school where they receive their Bachelor's in Science in Nursing (BSN). These programs are offered at universities. This path takes about four years to complete. After successfully completing the 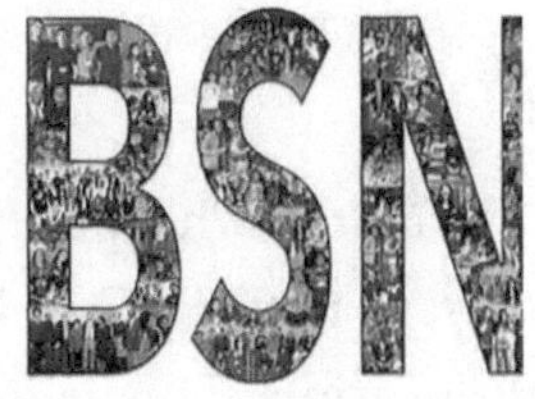 program, these students sit for the NCLEX and become Registered Nurses. The BSN-prepared nurse has more community nursing experience as well more management nursing experience, so they usually are well prepared to move into a leadership position at a nursing unit quickly.

Master of Science in Nursing (MSN): After one has received their nursing license and gained hands-on nursing experience for a few years, the option of receiving an MSN is a viable one. There are many 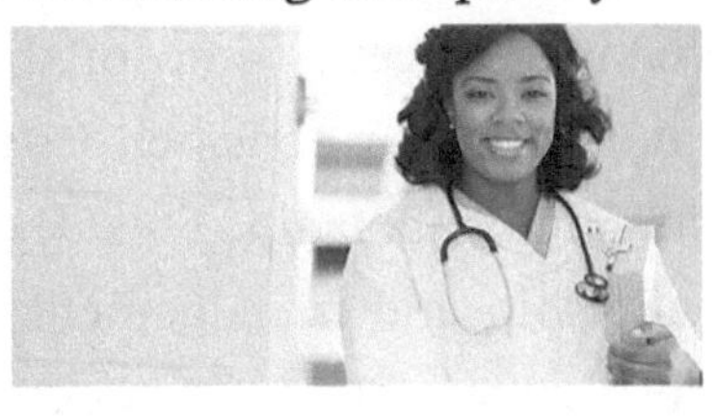 universities that offer online as well as onsite MSN programs. There are a variety of MSN programs available to nurses. There are MSN programs which prepare nurses to be Nurse Practitioners, Nurse Educators, or Nurse Leaders.

Nurse Practitioners are nurses who hold advanced degrees and can diagnose, prescribe, and treat patients. These nurses are trained in their area of specialty, either Family or Pediatrics, or Psychiatry to mention a few. They usually work with a medical doctor and have their own patient loads. This degree will take about two years to complete.

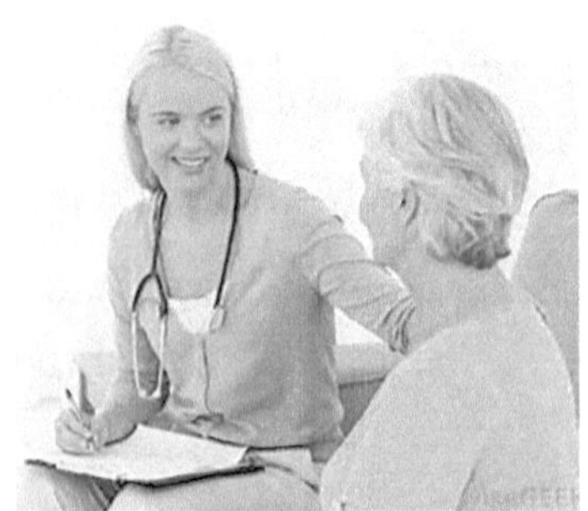
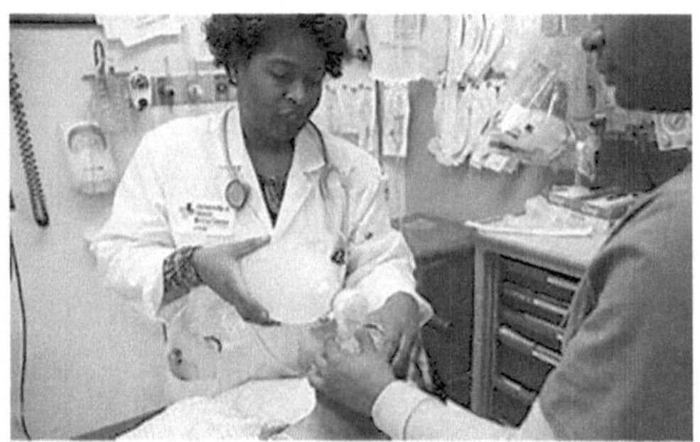

Nurse who have an interest in education might want to ultimately pursue their **PhD in Nursing Education** and choose the MSN in Nursing Education. This is a great steppingstone toward getting the PhD. These programs focus on nursing education and the theories of education and help develop your educational philosophies and teaching styles. This degree will take about two years to complete.

For nurses interested in becoming a Chief Nursing Officer of a hospital, or large medical group, one may consider getting their MSN in Nursing Leadership. This degree will focus on leadership and management skills needed for those career paths. This degree will take about two years to complete.

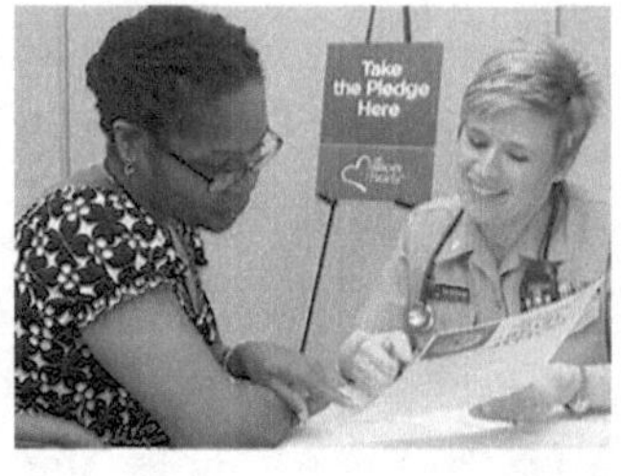

For those interested in becoming Nurse Practitioners you should know that not only is the MSN required, but now a **Doctor of Nursing Practice (DNP)** is highly encouraged as well. The DNP is a doctorate level education that prepares Nurse Practitioners to use the current evidence at the bedside. This degree teaches Nurse Practitioners the best way to bring the theory, research, and evidence to the patient at the bedside. This degree will take about three years to complete.

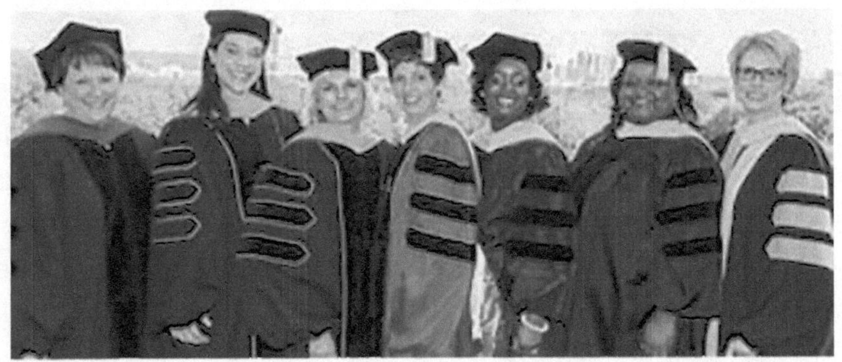

For those interested in the education route, a PhD in Nursing Education might be the way to go. For those interested in educational theory and research this is a perfect fit. Usually, people interested in a PhD in nursing education have goals of working in academia where the PhD is considered the terminal degree, and usually preferred for a nursing faculty. This degree will take about four years to complete.

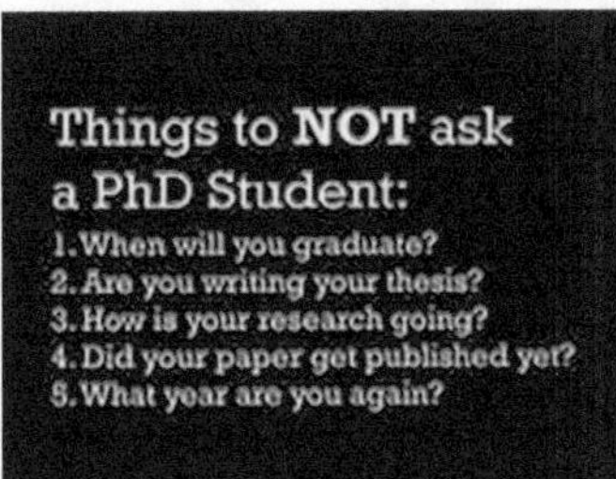

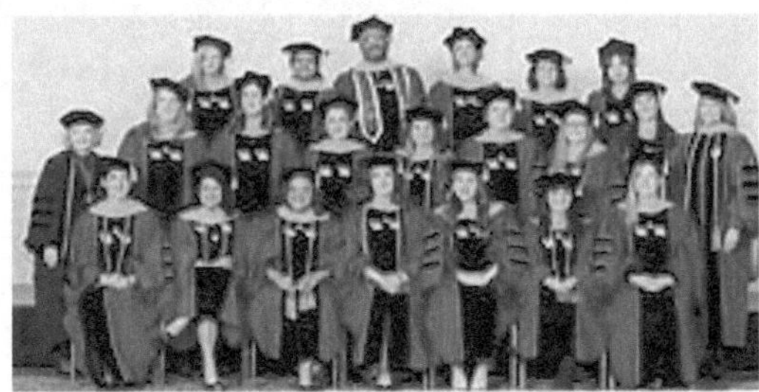

As you can see, graduating from an ASN/ADN or BSN program is just the beginning. There are many opportunities to continue with your education and specialize even more as you continue with your career. There is no "right "or "wrong" way to become a nurse. You have to decide which path is best for you and your career goals.

So, we have talked about the amazing opportunities waiting for you after you graduate. Let's recap what you can expect once you are in school.

WHAT CAN YOU EXPECT ONCE IN SCHOOL?

Long Hours and Hard Work:

As we have said before, nursing school is hard work. You should expect to spend many hours a day studying and preparing for your classes. It is advised not to work while going to nursing school. Many students apply for grants and scholarships so they can focus solely on school and be successful.

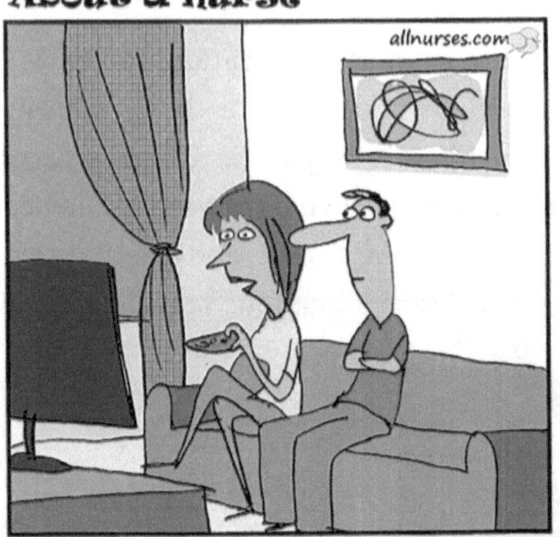

"I must spend a lot of time at the hospital, because I have over 1,200 shows recorded that I haven't watched."

Expect to spend three to nine hours preparing for EACH class. If you are taking four classes at a time that is 12 to 36 hours a week *preparing* for lecture. Most nursing classes have a clinical component associated with the lecture and most clinical rotations run between eight and twelve hours long. So, if you are taking four classes per week that is many hours a week preparing for the classes. Then you must attend class which will most likely be one to three hours per class. After class you can expect to study about three to five hours per class per week. Then you have your clinical hours. One exercise to do is the following:

Add up how many hours you spend a week on the following:

- Sleeping
- Eating meals
- Preparing meals
- Spending time with friends and family
- Working

Now factor in the above information based on three hours per class for preparation time, attending classes, studying and clinical rotations. Most people will find there is not any time left to work. The point is that working while attending nursing school is not advised. Something will suffer. It will either be your grades, or your work. Speaking about grades, most nursing schools have

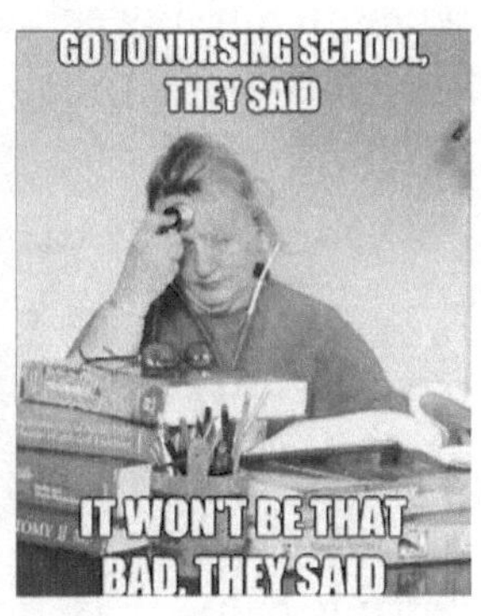

higher standards than general education in terms of "passing". Some schools set "passing" at 80% and some higher and some may be a few percentage points lower. You do not want to be a nurse who minimally passed nursing school. Nobody wants a nurse who only knows 75% of Medical Surgical nursing caring for them. The point is that going to nursing school is a commitment of time. You must put in the time to be successful.

Weird Hours:

We mentioned those clinical rotations. Clinical rotations are usually between eight and twelve hours long. Some schools have you go to the hospital the night before to get your patient assignments for the next day so you can prepare your nursing care plan the night before. Some clinicals may be on the weekends and some clinicals may begin at 6 am. Some clinicals may begin at 12 pm. It varies. The clinical placements are dependent upon your school, but the expectation is that you will attend every clinical each week. Most schools have policies such as missing more than one day of clinical in a semester is grounds for failure. Clinical rotation is not an option because it is in clinicals where you put the theory of your lectures into practice. People who work have a hard time rearranging their work schedule every semester around their clinical schedule for that semester as the clinical days and times usually change every semester, or term. So, our point is that when in nursing school, you must be flexible, you must be present, and you must be willing to sacrifice to be successful. You may miss family gatherings, or friend/social gatherings. You may not be able to go on the yearly family vacation. You may have to ask for help to ensure your family is taken care of. Remember the payout—all the opportunities that await you on the other side.

This brings us to another point: getting help. It is important that your family and friends know the sacrifices you will need to make to be successful in nursing school. It is important to have this conversation with them before you begin the program. You should schedule your childcare, errands, and grocery shopping ahead of time. You should ask for the support of your family and friends while you are in school. You should tell them what the expectations are of you while in the program so people are willing to step in and help you to be successful. The adjustment is

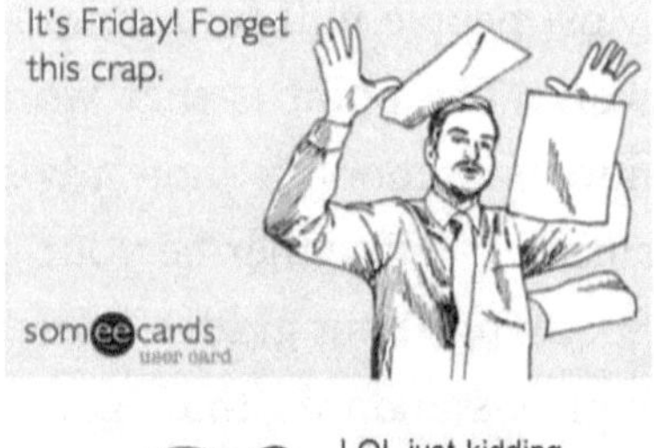

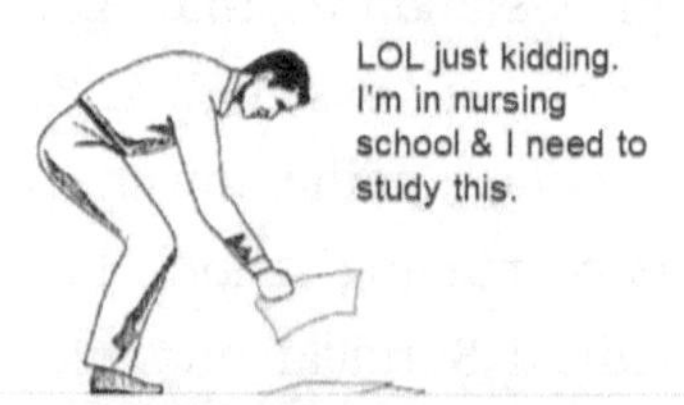

not only going to be hard for you, but for your friends and family as well. Make sure you have support and have people willing to help you in this endeavor.

You can expect to drive a lot while in nursing school. Usually, you will be at different hospitals during your nursing school experience. You should expect to have to have a working car and one that is reliable. You will be expected to be on time for your clinical so you must ensure your car is reliable and will get you to where you need to be. As mentioned above missing one clinical or being late to a clinical can result in the failure of a nursing class.

- Long hours
- Hard Work
- Weird Hours
- A lot of travel
- A lot of time away from home
- Classes and clinical
- Math tests
- About 80 to 90 hours a week of nursing school
- Really should not work
- Papers, presentations to classmates as well as agencies

GOALS

What are your goals in your future career in nursing?

You need to self-reflect and know your goals so you can make the correct actions to reach them.

HOW DO YOU SET GOALS?

Short term goals: Identify the steps necessary to get there (this is different for different people).

Long term goals: Identify what you want to do, or what you want to be first.

Identify your priorities in life and start planning your goals from there. Everyone's situation is different. Be realistic with your goals so you don't get disappointed if you don't reach them.

Write down a long-term goal and identify 5 short-term goals to reach that larger goal.

TIME MANAGEMENT

Time management is huge for nursing school. You will have multiples assignments due around the same time. You need to know yourself: When are you the most awake, when do you have the most energy?

Use whatever tools you need to reach your goals in a timely fashion: Calendar, notes, lists. PLAN AHEAD.

You need to factor in leisure time as well. This is time that allows you to regenerate and rejuvenate.

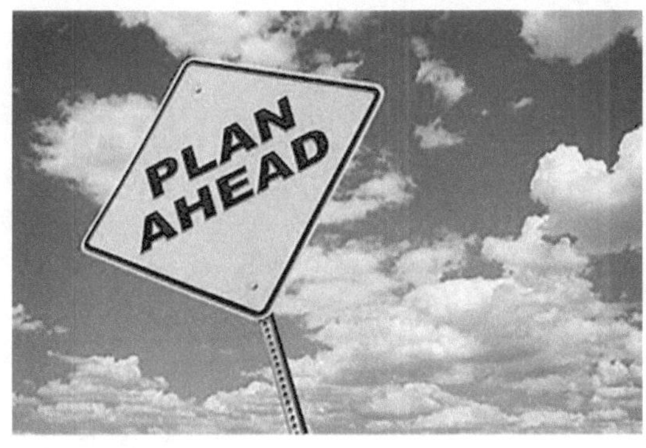

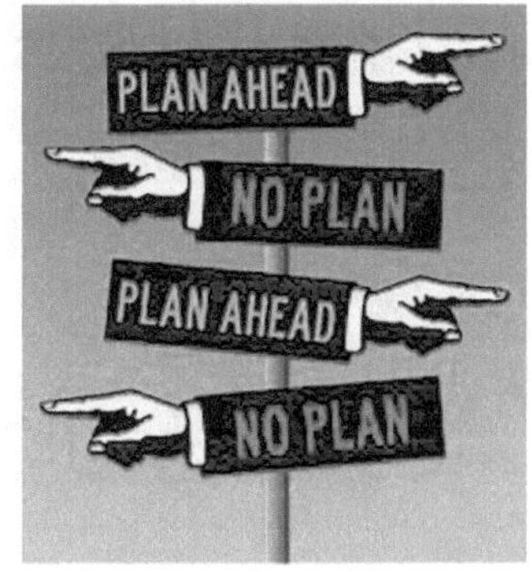

Things you should try hard to avoid
- Procrastination
- Perfectionism
- Fear of limitations: not sure if you have what it takes to do the job
- Being unsure of the next step: ASK QUESTIONS
- TO DO: Break projects into smaller goals along the way

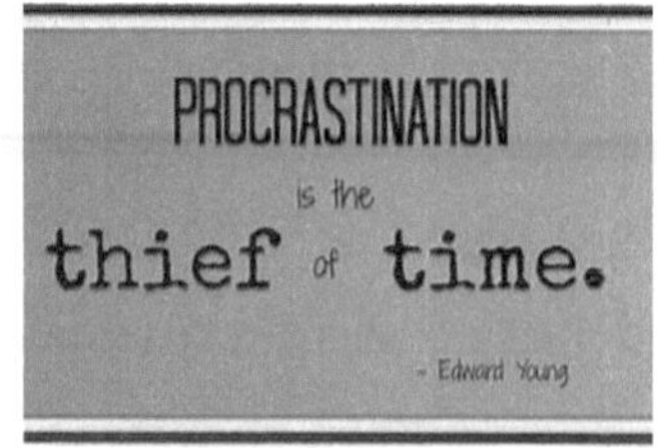

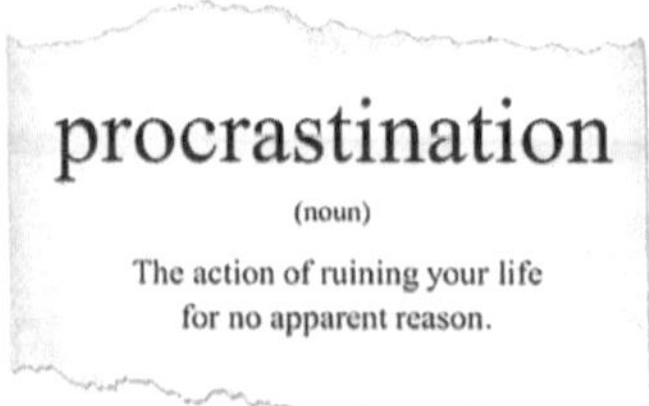

RELIEVING STRESS

How can you be a nursing student and relieve stress?

- Eat right
- Exercise
- Get sleep
- Seek balance
- Ask for help
- Learn to say "no" to more work

STRESS AND STRESS MANAGEMENT

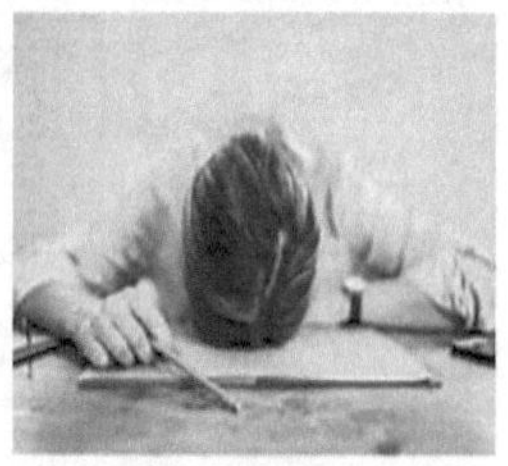
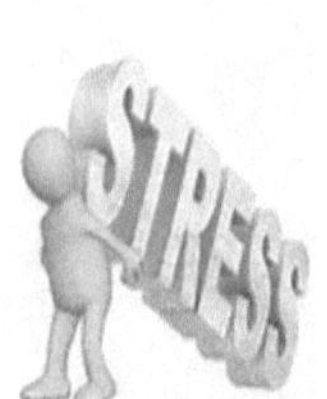

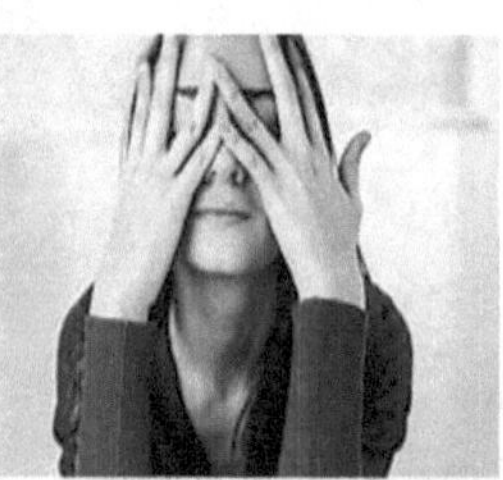

Nursing school will be a stressful time for you and your loved ones. You will miss out on family dinners, events, and maybe even trips! I know, it sounds painful, but it is only for a small amount of time in your life.

Even though nursing school will shoot up to the top of the list as the number one priority, make sure it is the number one priority when you are at school, clinical, or studying. You need time to move that priority down to number two or three when you are "off". There will be hundreds of pages to read, tests to prepare for, presentations to complete, and on and on, but remember you need to take care of YOU. Taking care of you looks different to everyone else. This might mean spending every Sunday afternoon from 1:00 pm to 6:00 pm with your family or friends. This might mean allowing yourself a massage or a manicure and pedicure once a month. Anything that is going to recharge your batteries is what you need to place in your schedule. Literally block this time off in your calendar and do what you need to do in that time. During this time, you are not going to think about, or worry about school. Know you will get back to it when your personal time is over. This is actually a great mindset to get into as a student because working nurses suffer from this too! Working nurses feel "bad" or "guilty" for not staying late after a shift or coming in on their day off to help! The truth is that you cannot take care of others unless you care for yourself first. Block out your personal time and stick to it. Your body and brain need this time out from school!

Stress: a condition or feeling experienced when a person perceives that demands exceed personal and social resources that the individual can mobilize.

It is what we feel when we lose control of our resources.

What are some stressors for you?

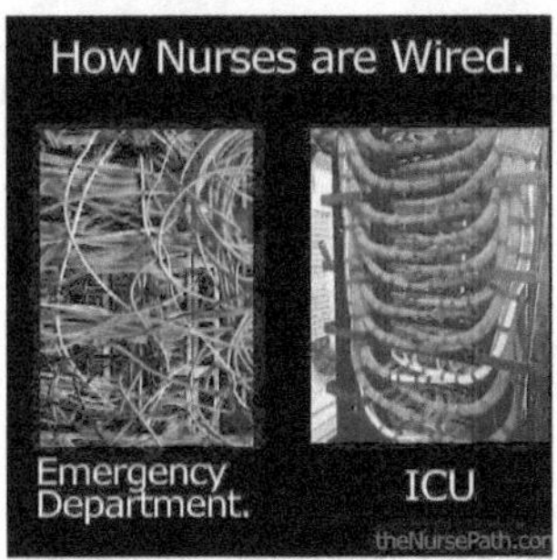

Common causes of stress: School, kids, jobs, spouses, time, or lack of time

Negative aspects of stress: frustration, irritability, depression, poor concentration, poor decision making, irrational beliefs, withdrawal, apprehension, fatigue, insomnia, self-medicating

Irrational beliefs: I should do everything without being stressed out; I have to please everyone by doing what is asked of me; I feel guilty if I take time for myself; I can't ask for help or I will feel like a failure.

Stress: 70-80% of MD visits are caused by stress-related symptoms

Stress: caused by stressors

Anxiety: stress that continues after the stressor is gone

How does stress affect us? You can get sick easier, suppression of immune system, and can cause hormonal imbalances.

Stress management: techniques people can use to deal with stress and lessen it

Managing stress: eat right, think positive, make a schedule, choose supportive people in your life, don't compare yourself to others, and don't use ETOH or drugs to deal with your issues.

Dealing with stress: Guided imagery, yoga, diet, breathing, get enough sleep, laugh, massage.

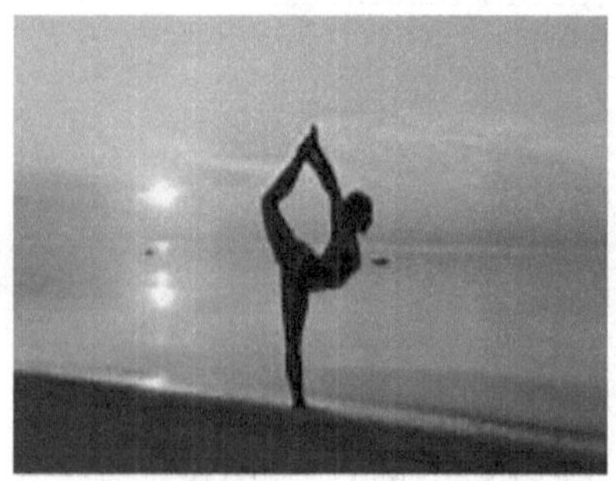
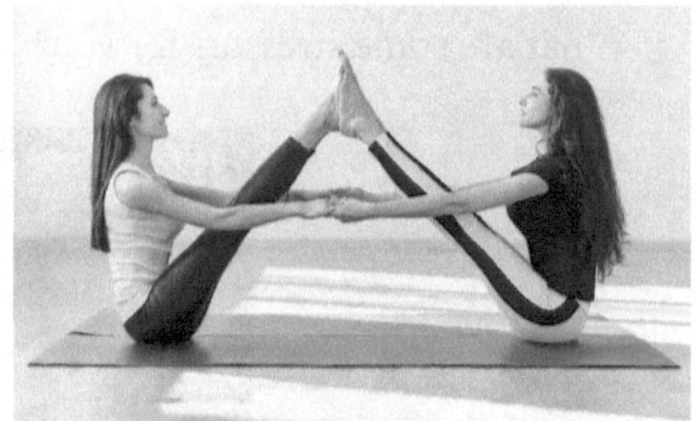

Foods to avoid: caffeine, sugar, chocolate, red meat, saturated fat. I had to put this in here but we all know coffee is a must and sometimes a donut is needed!

FINANCIAL AID

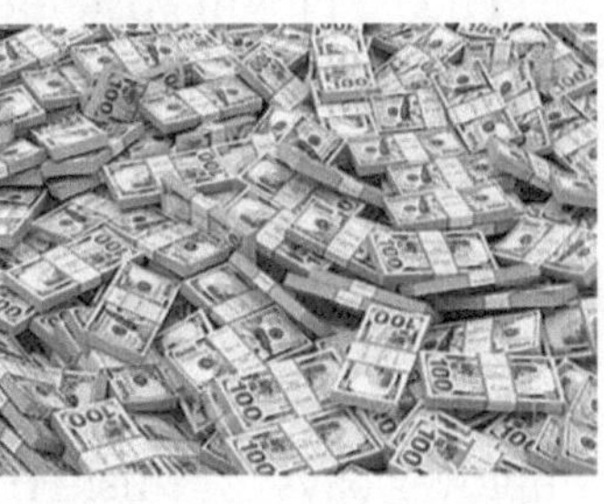

Yes, nursing school will cost money. Some nursing schools cost more than others, but they all cost money. This is something to think about when deciding which degree you want to pursue. If you start with an LPN program it will cost money to go back for the ASN/ADN program. If you start with the ASN.ADN program, it will cost money to go back for the BSN. If you start with the BSN program, it will cost money to go back for the MSN. You get the point!

Know what you want to spend and how you want to spend your money. Does it make more financial sense to go straight to the BSN, or does it make more sense to work your way up so you can work as an LPN to pay for the ASN/ADN? The choice is yours and nobody else's. Being an LPN is awesome. There are LPNs out there who know more than some physicians I know. However, if you plan to continue with your education when will this be? How much money will you take out of each paycheck to put aside for future schooling? The reason I am asking these questions is because it is HARD to go back to school once you graduate. Make a list of your goals and make a plan to reach those goals. I am not going to lie, after graduating you start making money, you don't have homework, you don't have projects to do, and it is nice to get "settled". You can take a break from school. Go on vacation, go to family dinners, have fun, and then get back to your goal list!

What costs money? Everything.

School is one more bill to add to the pile.

Credit cards: sounds like a great way to pay for things now, but try not to build up a lot of debt before starting school because school is expensive, and you don't need to be worried about how to pay the credit card bills on top of tuition and cost of living

The LPN will cost you about $10,000 to $12,0000

The ADN can cost you about $15,000 to $30,0000

The BSN can cost you between 20,000 and 80,000 dollars

The MSN, DNP and PhD will run another $10,000 each

You will be required to take continuing education every year for your nursing license, and this will run about $500.00 a year (unless your employer pays for this! HINT, HINT!!)

On top of tuition, you will need to pay for:

Gas, parking fees, ATI fees, uniforms, CPR, a physical exam, immunizations, TB test, a drug screen, background check, application for graduation, NCLEX fee, license fee, fingerprints.

The rule of thumb is to have 6 months of all bills saved in case of a rainy day!

Where can I Find Money?

FAFSA (Government loan FAFSA.gov)

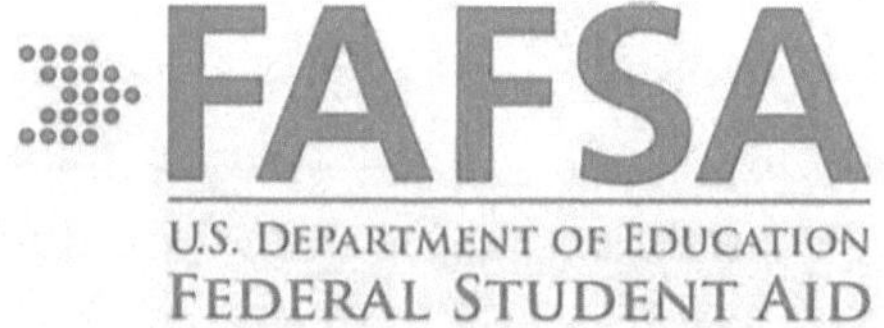

HRSA (A great government resource)

Grants through school, scholarships: After you graduate you can apply for student loans to be forgiven if you work in certain areas. Always check the HRSA website as they are always giving nurses breaks on their financial aid due!

The truth is there is money out there for students, especially nursing students. Take an afternoon and search which grants or scholarships you qualify for and apply! If you don't receive a grant or a scholarship right off the bat, keep applying, keep asking, and keep searching! New money seems to pop up each year for nurses. There are even "financial aid forgiveness" programs for nurses after graduating. Some facilities might pay your tuition if you sign a contract to work for them for X number of years. If you look hard enough, you will find money!

Learning styles: Different approaches or ways of learning

We talked about this when we discussed nursing school above. Here are some examples:

Types of learning styles: Visual, tactile, auditory

Visual Learners: Remember what you read, you enjoy visual projects, and remember charts, graphs, and maps.

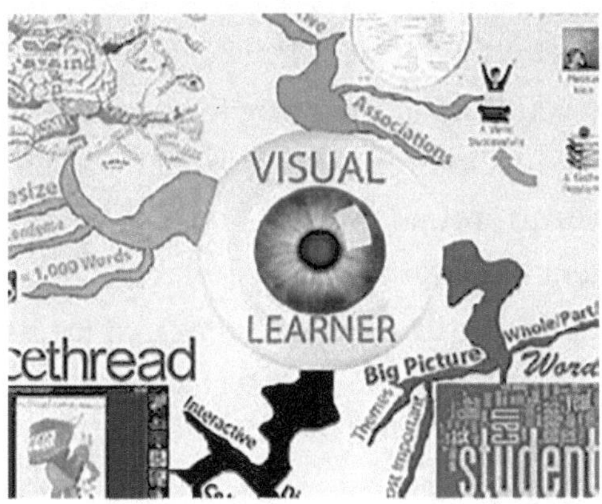

Learning strategies for visual learners:
- Work in a quiet place
- Learn alone
- Take many notes
- Re write and re write notes
- Use color highlights
- Before reading a chapter, scan it for pictures/charts
- Use flashcards
- Use posters, videos

Tactile learners: Remembers what they do, enjoys active participation, has good motor coordination.

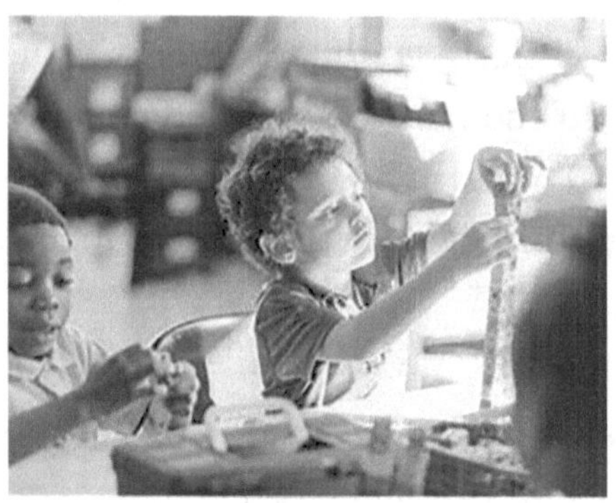

Learning strategies for tactical learners:
- Pace or walk around while using flashcards
- Try studying in a lounge chair or a bean bag chair
- Study with background music
- Take frequent breaks
- Try learning by picturing words/ideas/concepts in your head

Auditory learners: Remembers what they hear, enjoys classroom and small discussions.

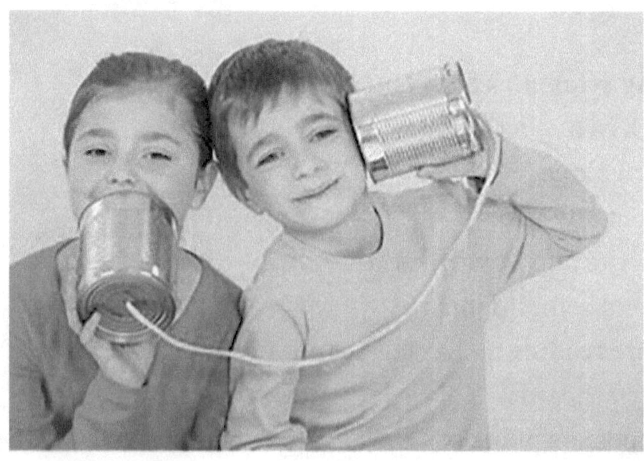

Learning strategies for auditory learners:
- Recite the information out loud
- Ask to do oral presentations instead of written
- Make tapes of important points and listen to them over and over
- Make flashcards using different colors
- Set goals and verbalize them
- Read out loud
- HEAR the words as you read

Which type of learning style do you most enjoy and why?
- Lecture
- Group discussion
- Small group
- Visual focus
- Verbal focus
- Logical presentation
- Random presentation

How much do we really remember?
- 5% from lecture
- 10% from reading
- 20% from visual graphs
- 30% demonstration
- 50% discussion groups
- 75% practice doing
- 90% teaching others

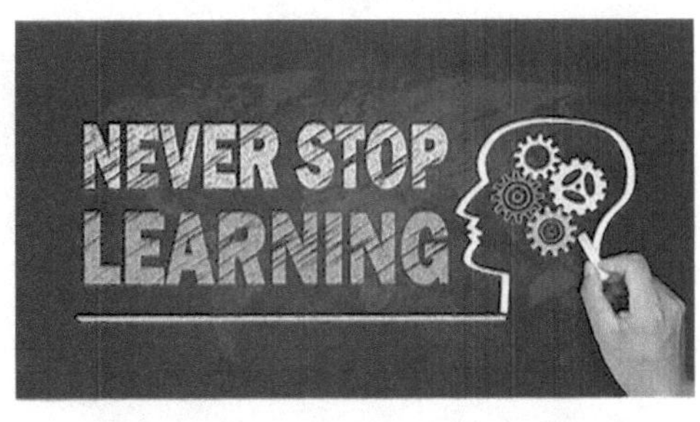

YOU CAN DO THIS AND WE WILL WELCOME YOU INTO THE PROFESSION WITH OPEN ARMS!

Quotes from nurses in the workforce who are on your side and cheering you on from the sidelines:

Always think of your resident as if it was your family you are treating.
Judy Moore

Always try to put yourself in the patient's position and react accordingly. It's not easy being the patient and being scared or hurt, sometimes they react in a not so pleasant way. Before you react or speak back think about how you may would feel.
Jessica Bonner Moore

I am not sure if you are interested in a quote from a nurse who just celebrated her 40th nursing anniversary. But to me the most important thing new nurses can carry with them through the years is the value of mentoring at every opportunity and supporting each other every day.
Ilene Rusnak

Can I say to always trust your gut instinct.
Don't be afraid to speak up or ask a question.
Karla M

Never let Your Nursing license expire, always renew.
Lisa Harrison

Be prepared to give your all and learn that it is okay to ask questions!
Kylie Hood

Challenge every wrong question. Whether it's to learn why you got it wrong, or to prove you got it right, challenge every wrong question.
Matthew Harville RN

Dare to love and become a pediatric nurse.
Branden Murphy RN

*Learn to stand for what you believe is true,
either for a procedure or an examination question.
You keep learning in nursing; nursing is more about on-the-job training.*
Daramola Abisola RN

Having a substance abuse patient do 30 more days because I was his nurse
Donald Orlan

*Always remember that we were once new grads.
Take the time to teach and help each other grow.*
Lorena Ortiz-Hernandez

Listen to your patients. More times than not, they can help avert a mistake.
Michelle Forbes

It was my clinical rotation at student life, when gunshot patient cried on my shoulder, for the first time I felt blessed, and those tears helped me a lot whenever I felt exhausted in workplace even after student life.
Karim Dad

It's important to remember that often times, as bedside nurses we are interacting with our patients and their families at some of the hardest and scariest points in their lives. Something that is just another day at work for us can be scary and traumatizing for them. Be patient, understanding and kind. Don't forget the importance and significance of educating your patient and their family about what is happening around them.
Abigail Anderson

Nursing is absolutely the best profession. There are so many things you can do as a registered nurse! From providing direct care at the bedside, using sharp clinical assessment skills and the tools of technology; to quality improvement and data analysis; to case management, to utilization management where your clinical skills are used as part of the revenue cycle. The possibilities are endless. The absolute best profession that allows you to demonstrate the art of caring in collaboration with the science of technology!
Lauren Pond, RN

Never forget the "why". Why did I become a nurse? When you always keep the "why" in view, it will help you make it through the challenges of nursing.
Laura Marovich

As a nurse, it's better to be a leader. However, it's best to be the dealer. In a true sense, you should be able to deal proficiently not only with living beings of all kinds but also with emerging trends and advanced technology.
Sonia, RN, MSN

No matter your degree or initials after your name, you are never too good to answer a call bell, comfort a patient, or change a bedpan. Stay humble and remember why you became a nurse
Renee Newberry

Nursing can take you anywhere and you can work in many specializations or have a career in just one. The choice is yours, just don't give up!
Sue Hogan

Nursing is versatile, the road is endless! Find your happiness.
Ashley Leach

The best part of nursing is holding someone's hand as they leave this world and knowing they were not alone at the end of their life!
Karen Valdez RN for 25 years

"If you didn't succeed, it's just as important to keep in mind that there has never been a success story without failure and lessons along the way, failing the exams 2 times made me want to give up but the failures taught me lessons and I never gave up so I passed in my third attempt, inbox me if you want to know how I made it through my exams I'd be happy to help out
Yaouba Salli

A tool has been created by the author of this book to help nursing students integrate and synthesize all the information nursing students will need to safely care for patients. The tool is called NurseMuse.

Check it out at www.nursemuse.com

The tool is a handy one that will allow you to link the medical diagnoses to the nursing diagnoses to the interventions to the rationale. It also serves as a one-stop-shop for resources you need while caring for patients!

Here is an article about the tool!

A handy resource – breaking news!

A BETTER CARE PLAN: NURSEMUSE

By Joseph Gaccione

Intro

UNLV Nursing alumna Catherine Prato-Lefkowitz didn't set out to invent something for nursing. But thanks to a conversation with a pharmacy executive, she now oversees a new brand she hopes will ease a nursing student's education.

Three years ago, Prato-Lefkowitz conceptualized a digital program that would alleviate nursing student anxiety called NurseMuse. This program would store all necessary and relevant information for students building care plans for patients into one centralized space.

NurseMuse launched officially Spring 2022 with the twin goals of simplifying both nurse notetaking and erasing any ambiguity about what a care plan is.

Background

Prato-Lefkowitz came up with NurseMuse as a graduate student at UNLV, but despite earning three nursing degrees, it actually started in a non-health care field. She explains the idea started while studying for her Executive MBA at UNLV. She was brainstorming ideas for a thesis in her entrepreneurship class. It was during a conversation with other business leaders she realized what that could be. She recalled, "When I was talking to CVS, their CEO said, 'I don't know how nurses keep track of all those notes, writing all this stuff down throughout the day. That must be cumbersome.' I said, 'Yes, it's called the nursing brain board. We just take a piece of paper and all of our patients [are] written down. That's when it clicked that I could incorporate this into nursing education and help students understand the 'why.'"

But the idea evolved further from just notetaking. Prato-Lefkowitz realized she could build something that emphasized the purpose of what students were trying to achieve. "The nursing faculty would tell students, 'At the end, it's going to come together.' When I was a student, I was like, 'I don't know what is supposed to come together,'" Prato-Lefkowitz says. "So, you're a new nurse, stuck in the hospital. You have patients with diagnoses, and you don't know what the diagnoses are. Then you're told you have to write a care plan based on your nursing and medical diagnoses. That's very overwhelming."

Additionally, Prato-Lefkowitz made sure to always keep the "why" at the top of her priority list. When she asks her students why they perform a task, she wants a well-thought-out response. "I need an evidence-based rationale answer instead of, 'We have a doctor's order.' We don't do that anymore," she explains. "It's all evidence-based practice." She added, "I can make it easier for our students to see the whole package upfront and then try to peel back the layers."

Building the program

Although Prato-Lefkowitz has extensive nursing experience, transferring her knowledge into a program wasn't easy. For her, it was like being a freshman student. "I feel I went through nursing school again after putting it together," she admits. "I probably have 250-300 diagnoses in the care plan right now you can link, but I hand wrote all those. I used my evidence and textbooks. I had to research." Additionally, she found a programmer in India to help with the actual software building. When NurseMuse was ready to test, she shared the program with UNLV nursing students to get their take on what works and what could be improved. "I'd say, 'Tell me what's missing.' They say, 'It would be great if we could pull up normal vital signs for a baby versus an elderly patient,' or 'It would be great to look up a normal lab value.' It started evolving from there, getting feedback from nursing students," Prato-Lefkowitz says. The more responses she received, the more comprehensive the care plans became.

NurseMuse was built during the height of COVID-19, when Prato-Lefkowitz was also working as a nurse. But she argues the pandemic helped her focus more on the program, specifically for possible future shutdowns that limit clinical resources for students. "A lot of students never entered a hospital. Now, they're graduating nurses, and they've never touched a patient," she says. "I think with this program, we can use it with simulation or case study, or integrate it into our curriculum so our students get more of that understanding, which is important for how these concepts connect with one another. Then, if they don't get to touch a patient, at least they're going to understand that 'why.'"

Program Facts

The NurseMuse interface divides its resources into useful tabs for either a nursing student or a registered nurse. Information accessible includes medical and nursing diagnoses; vital sign ranges, medical terminology; labs; and more, all evidence-based and referenced. "There are a ton of resources there," Prato-Lefkowitz explains. "If I'm a nursing student, and I forgot what the normal value of hemoglobin is, I can look it up on NurseMuse. I can also document everything for my patient that day. I can create the care plan, print it out and turn it in to my professor. It's very HIPAA-compliant; only I can access my patients I've put in."

One of the distinctions in NurseMuse is between nursing and medical diagnoses. Prato-Lefkowitz explains nurses cannot solely use a medical diagnosis because of the different areas of practice and different objectives between physicians and nurses. She adds there are both medical problems and nursing problems, requiring different interventions for each. "We don't treat hypertension. We treat decreased cardiac output, because we're nurses and we have to have a special language," she says. "We aren't treating the medical diagnosis, which is challenging for our nursing students to understand. I have a patient who has hypertension. They have high blood pressure, but we aren't treating the high blood pressure. Our physician is treating the high blood pressure by ordering these medications. We're going to give them medications, but we as nurses have to understand how those medications work in our system and look for any adverse effects or any positive or negative outcomes."

Additional technological resources in nursing (or health care, in general) is a commonality these days, and Prato-Lefkowitz wants to stick to the modern trend to keep up with our future nurses. "I think our students these days are used to growing up with their computer. When I was in nursing school, we would be at home with our textbooks, finding nursing diagnoses. But now, our students are used to opening a link and having everything at their fingertips, which I think is important because that's how it's going to be when they graduate and become practicing nurses." However, she says there can always be a risk to relying too heavily on technology. "When we teach how to take blood pressure, we teach [students] how to manually take blood pressure with the stethoscope and [cuff]," she says. "Our students say, 'I don't know why [we're doing manual], because we have automatic [machines] in the hospitals.' What if your automatic one isn't working, or what if there's an emergency or what if your provider asks for a manual on both sides?" She adds, "You have to understand our foundation. With NurseMuse, I'm trying to teach them that foundation. It's great if they use it. But if it's not working correctly, hopefully from their prior history of using it, they should already know what they're looking for with the patient. If they can't access it, it should not be the end of the world."

Feedback and Future

NurseMuse launched three months ago, and Prato-Lefkowitz is spreading more awareness about her program. Her overall goal is to implement the program in nursing schools across the country. Currently, Prato-Lefkowitz has been in talks with eight schools in Nevada, including UNLV, before shifting her focus to California and other regions. Long-term, she also wants to expand NurseMuse for certified nursing assistants and nurse practitioners.

She acknowledges there is much to learn about the business side of introducing a new product, specifically marketing. "I believe with any new system, you just have to hear it: 'NurseMuse, NurseMuse', and eventually somebody will say, 'Maybe I should check it out.' We're in that phase of just trying to get it out there. It's grassroots right now, but I'm going to keep promoting it."

One particular review convinced Prato-Lefkowitz she was heading in the right direction. "I showed this to a nurse at Henderson Hospital. He's an ICU nurse, ex-military, going to med school. He said, 'This is the most awesome thing I've ever seen. This could be huge.' I thought, 'He's a smart dude. He used to do IVs in a helicopter, and I have his blessing. At least I'm not wasting my time.'"